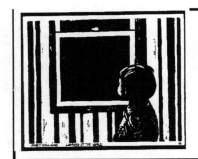

THE MORNING NEWS

Carol Gray, Editor
Jenison Public Schools, Jenison, Michigan

Domestic and International Subscription Form

THE MORNING NEWS is a quarterly newsletter that informally shares practical information among parents and professionals working on behalf of children and adults with autism and related disorders. Articles address a wide variety of concerns, and share ideas which update and expand the use of social stories and related techniques and materials.

THE MORNING NEWS is available directly from Jenison Public Schools. To subscribe, complete this form and return it to us with your check, money order or purchase order to the address below.

THE MORNING NEWS makes a wonderful gift for professionals and family: If this is a gift, a gift announcement will be sent. Check the gift box in the subscription form below and indicate how the card should be signed in the space provided in the square below.

Subscription rates for one year : U.S. Subscriptions = $18.00 U.S.
Canada and Mexico= $20.00 U.S.   All other countries=$22.00 U.S.

Please print or type

Name_____Phone (optional)_____

Complete Address_____

_____

Zip Code (if applicable)_____Country_____

Please check the appropriate space: ___New   ___Renewal   ___Gift - please
sign   gift   card   as   follows:_____

Send completed form along with payment to:

THE MORNING NEWS   **Phone:**   **616-457-8955**
Carol Gray, Editor   **FAX:**   **616-457-8442**
Jenison High School
2140 Bauer Road
Jenison, Michigan   49428

Thank You!

All marketing and publishing rights guaranteed to and reserved by:
Future Horizons, Inc. 721 W. Abram St., Arlington, TX 76013
Tel: 800-489-0727; 817-277-0727; 817-277-2270 Fax
Website: www.FutureHorizons-autism.com   E-mail:edfuture@onramp.net

Address all correspondence to: Carol Gray, Consultant to Students with Autism,
Jenison High School, 2140 Bauer Road, Jenison, MI 49428.
Telephone: (616) 457-8955   Fax: (616) 457-4070

ISBN #1-885477-21-x

Taming the Recess JuNgle

Carol Gray
Consultant to Students with Autism
Jenison Public Schools

Cover design by Carol Gray

"Taming the Recess JuNgLe"

is a collection of materials to socially simplify recess.

In the fall of 1993, an article appeared in THE MORNING NEWS, a newsletter of Jenison Public Schools, titled, *That JuNgle We Call Recess*. This article discussed the social challenges of recess, and identified a variety of resources and materials to use to socially simplify recess for children with autism and related disorders.

This packet contains the article:

That JuNgLe We Call Recess

In addition, the materials referred to in the article
are included in this booklet in the following order:

Social Cues Questionnaire

The Sixth Sense

Socially Simplifying Recess with a Piece of Chalk

Sample Recess Social Story

That JuNgLe We Call "Recess"

Carol Gray
Consultant to Students with Autism
Jenison Public Schools

Twenty or so children are reading silently in their classroom. A bell rings. Suddenly desk tops fly open and shut in a pattern which defies any union or logic. Pencils fall to the floor. Children move to the door and papers fall from counters to mark their passing. In record preparation time that would put an army infantry to shame, a playground is suddenly filled with 534 children. Squirrels suspend efforts to gather nuts and birds decide to fly south. It's time for recess.

To a child with a disorder on the autistic spectrum, the confusion is only beginning. There are fifteen to thirty eternal minutes to go. Longer than it takes to read this article. Longer than it takes to load a dishwasher. To a child with autism, longer than it takes to do just about anything. As one child describes, "The problem with recess is all the children are free." In the words of another child, "Recess is when I am supposed to have fun and my teacher says 'Go outside and have fun'...but I don't."

The safest place in any jungle would seem to be on its fringes, and as a consultant, that is where I often find my students. If my students are not on the physical fringes of a playground, they are often on its social fringes. Many children with autism would like to play with others, but are seemingly lost and struggling to find direction in a land without signs or arrows. We've some ideas for those children which may help.

First, remember that the social struggle we may observe in children with autism at recess is not the problem - it is a result of the problem. The fact that s/he is often excluded is not the problem - it is also the result of the problem. Therefore, we need to take time to identify the problem from the perspective of the child with autism, *and* from that of other children. Asking the child with autism questions found in the recess section of The Social Cues Questionnaire may yield insights. Talking with other children at recess can also be informative. It's important to "know the jungle" before you attempt to "advise all the wildlife."

Once you understand recess, improving the understanding children have of their classmate with autism may be helpful. Talk with the classmates of the child with autism, explaining the challenges that child faces. One idea we have which is proving effective (based on informal feedback from teachers) is a presentation and class exercise which demonstrates what it's like to have difficulty with social skills. After briefly reviewing the five senses, this presentation identifies social ability as "The Sixth Sense." A class exercise follows which demonstrates how our "sixth" social sense works for us.

Often parents and professionals will express concern that "all the children tease" the child with autism. It's important to *accurately* identify the problem, as most likely only a few children are teasing. Try taking time to understand the child who is teasing. Considering teasing is viewed as insensitive and cruel, the temptation is to remind the aggressors of "how you would feel if you were being teased." They probably already *know* how they would feel, and may be looking for someone to acknowledge *their* feelings. While correction is in order, so is understanding, and an intervention based on understanding yields better results long term.

In addition, children who are teased need assistance to learn how to respond. Try beginning with "pencil and paper solutions" to real life teasing. For example, for a child who needs assistance to identify the "good guys" from the others on the playground, make two lists on a piece of paper. On one list are the children who ask "you to do things that you know are silly, or not right." In the other list, are children "who never ask you to do those things." One child saw the two lists and, taking the pencil from my hand, crossed off the children who were giving him trouble and announced, "There, they're gone." Once he had control of them on paper, he wrote down some solutions that he thought might "cross them off" at recess. The idea is to structure the discussion while providing visual feedback, enabling the child to determine his/her own solution.

A piece of chalk (or outdoor paints) may help to simplify a playground. Use these materials to add some visual, social structure to recess. For example, use chalk to create "waiting boxes" for a turn shooting baskets, with students walking from the last box to the first for a turn. Or, write playground rules on the blacktop. Identify for a student where to line up by writing the student's name in chalk on the pavement (others may want to write their name, too).

Depending on the student and situation, social stories may be effective for a variety of recess challenges. Remember to begin by taking the perspective of the child. Photographs have been used successfully in recess stories, describing each of the basic activities and equipment, thus "taking apart" a situation which may be overwhelming as a whole.

Pamela J. Wolfberg, Ph.D. has developed Integrated Play Groups to assist children as they learn to play with others. The purpose is to guide children with autism and related social-communicative needs (novice players) to play in both social and imaginative ways with typically developing peers (expert players). (For more information on Integrated Play Groups, visit www.integratedplaygroups.com or call 415-753-5669. Wolfberg's book "Play and Imagination in Children with Autism" is also available from Future Horizons, Inc.)

Another idea comes from Holmes Elementary School in Spring Lake, Michigan. An "outdoor classroom" with a seating area has been designated as a reading area on the playground. Students can take books outside and read during recess. This provides children who may not want to swing or play baseball with another free time option.

The recess bell rings and the process reverses. That social phenomenon known as recess comes to an end. The children return to their seats. By visually assisting our students through a variety of activities, the hope is that we can make "the jungle we call recess" more accessible and successful for children with disorders on the autistic spectrum.

Social Cues Questionnaire

Suggestions for Implementation

Carol Gray
Consultant for Students with Autism

The Social Cues Questionnaire is an informal checklist which can assist in identifying where a child is having difficulty in following the classroom routine and/or identifying, interpreting, and/or responding to social cues. These suggestions are intended guidelines, along with consideration of each child's learning style.

Select question which are the most relevant to the child's needs. One or two questions from each section may be selected, or an entire section.

It may be helpful to type the question onto a computer disc, enabling the child to directly respond to the questions independently. Or, for children who are unable to type, sit with the child at the computer, presenting each question in enlarged font. The child can dictate his/her response, focusing his /her attention on the computer screen which presents a visual display or your questions, and his/her answers.

It may also be helpful to use a small laminate marker board and markers to illustrate questions as they are presented. To do this, quickly draw stick figures to illustrate each question. This may improve the child's comprehension of your questions, enabling the child to respond more accurately.

Review a child's answers with the classroom teacher. A child may provide answers which appear logical and correct, though they may be inaccurate in terms of the current teacher's teaching style. For example, a child may report that his teacher turns off the lights when she wants the children to be quiet. It is important to share this response with the child's teacher, to make sure that the child is reporting what is currently true, vs. the behavior of a teacher from a previous grade. Reviewing a child's answers with the current classroom teacher ensures the answers you receive are accurate for the child's current classroom experience.

Social Cues Questionnaire

Name:_____ Date:_____

School:_____ Teacher:_____

The Morning Routine

1.   What is the first thing you should do when you get to school in the morning?

_____
_____
_____
_____

2.   When you finish that, what's next?

_____
_____
_____
_____
_____

3.   How do you know when it is time to stop doing that (#2)?

_____
_____
_____
_____
_____

4.   The hardest thing about starting the day at school is_____?

_____
_____
_____
_____

Rules

5.   Are there rules for the children in your class?

_____
_____
_____
_____
_____

6.   Are the rules up in the room? If so, where?

_____
_____
_____
_____
_____

7.   What rules can you remember?

_____
_____
_____
_____
_____

8.   Why do the children in your class have those rules?

_____
_____
_____
_____

9.   Which rule do you think is the best (*or* most important)?

_____
_____
_____
_____

10.   What rule do *you think* your class should have?

_____
_____
_____
_____

11.   One thing you should NEVER do in my class is_____.

_____
_____
_____
_____

12.   Does your class have a rule about raising your hand? If so, when do children raise their hand? (Why?)

_____
_____
_____
_____

13.   If you raise your hand to answer your teacher's question, will your teacher always call on you to give the answer?

_____
_____
_____
_____

My Teacher

My teacher's name is:_____

13.   How do you know when your teacher is talking just to you?
      How do you know when your teacher is talking to all the children at the same
      time?

      _____
      _____
      _____
      _____

14.   How do you know if your teacher is happy? (What does your teacher do? What
      does your teacher say?)

      _____
      _____
      _____
      _____

15.   How do you know when your teacher is angry? (What does your teacher do?
      What does your teacher say?)

      _____
      _____
      _____
      _____

16.   What is one thing that makes your teacher angry?

      _____
      _____
      _____
      _____

17.   How do you know when your teacher is going to say something REALLY
       important? (What does your teacher do? What does your teacher say?)

_____
_____
_____
_____

18.   How do you know when your teacher is joking or teasing (trying to make others
       laugh)? (What does your teacher do? What does your teacher say?)

_____
_____
_____
_____

17.   My teacher likes it when children_____.

_____
_____
_____
_____

18.   What does your teacher do when it is time for a lesson to begin?

_____
_____
_____
_____

19.   One thing my teacher does that I really like is_____

_____
_____
_____
_____
_____

Lines

20.   When do all the children in your class walk in a line?

_____
_____
_____
_____

21.   Why do you think teachers ask children to walk in lines?

_____
_____
_____
_____

22.   How do you know when you should get in a line with the other children?
       (What does your teacher say? What does your teacher do?)

_____
_____
_____
_____

23.   What does it feel like to *stand* in a line?

_____
_____
_____
_____

24.   Do you like standing and walking in lines at school? (Why or why not?)

_____
_____
_____

25.   Who gets to be first in line?

_____
_____
_____
_____

26.   How do you know who gets to be first in line?

_____
_____
_____
_____

27.   Would you like to be first in line, at the end of the line, or somewhere in between?

_____
_____
_____
_____

28.   What should a child do if it is time to get in line and they are not finished with their work?

_____
_____
_____
_____

29.   Does your class ever line up outside?

_____
_____
_____
_____

Recess

30.   Tell me about recess.

_____
_____
_____
_____

31.   How do you know when it is time for recess?

_____
_____
_____
_____

32.   What do you like to do at recess?

_____
_____
_____
_____

33.   What are some things other children do at recess?

_____
_____
_____
_____

34.   What should you do if it's time for recess and you haven't finished your work?

_____
_____
_____
_____

35.   Are there rules at recess? If so, what are some of the rules?

_____
_____
_____
_____

36.   What do you think is the best thing about recess?

_____
_____
_____
_____

37.   Is there anything about recess you don't like? Can you tell me about it?

_____
_____
_____
_____

38.   What is the funniest thing you have ever seen at recess?

_____
_____
_____
_____

39.   How do you know when it is time to come in from recess?

_____
_____
_____
_____

Getting Help

40. How does your teacher know when you need help?

_____
_____
_____
_____

41. If a child in your class needs help, what should they do?

_____
_____
_____

42. Everyone needs help sometimes. When do you think you need help?

_____
_____
_____

43. What things can you do to help children in your class?

_____
_____
_____
_____

44. Which people in your class can help you if you need it?

_____
_____
_____
_____

Transitions

45. What is the first thing you usually do after the morning recess?

_____
_____
_____

46. What is the first thing you usually do after lunch?

_____
_____
_____

47. What is the first thing you usually do after the afternoon recess?

_____
_____
_____

48. Where do children put papers that they finish?

_____
_____
_____

49. If a child in your class finished ALL of their work, what can they do?

_____
_____
_____

Friends and Classmates

50. What does the word *friend* mean?

_____
_____
_____

51. A friend is someone who...

_____
_____
_____

52. Do you have a friend in your class? What is your friend's name?

_____
_____
_____

53. What do people mean when they ask, "Have you made any friends?"

_____
_____
_____
_____
_____

54. Many of the children in my class like ... (name of a classmate)

_____
_____
_____

55. The reason so many children like _(from answer to #54)__ is...

_____
_____
_____

56. If I want to play with someone, here's what I do....

_____
_____
_____

57. One thing I like to do with other children is....

_____
_____

58. Each child likes to do different things. Here is a list of ten things children like to do:

1._____ 6._____
2._____ 7._____
3._____ 8._____
4._____ 9._____
5._____ 10._____

59. One thing my friend likes to do is...

_____
_____

60. A "best friend" is...

_____
_____
_____

The Sixth Sense
Lesson Plan: For use with students ages 8 - 18+

-Carol Gray
Consultant to Students with Autism

Goal: To improve general education students' understanding of disorders on the autistic spectrum, especially in the areas of communication and social cognition which directly impact on general education students.

To support and guide general education students as they determine effective means to assist their classmate with a disorder on the autistic spectrum.

Objective(s):   Students will review the five senses and discuss: (1) their role in gathering information, (2) whether senses are learned or "automatic", and (3) the result of impairments in selected senses (hearing, sight).

Students will participate in a demonstration which illustrates how people "automatically" keep track of what other people perceive, think, and feel.

Students will learn why our social sense may be considered a "sixth sense" by comparing our ability to acquire and process social information with how information is acquired and processed via the other senses.

Students will identify possible results of an impairment in our social sense.

Students will identify effective means to assist a classmate with a disorder on the autistic spectrum.

Materials: Small item to hide (stuffed animal)
Chalkboard or laminate marker board

Procedure: *Introduction: Explain to the class that you will/are going to help them understand their classmate, _____.* Explain that you are going to demonstrate to the class, in part, what it might be like if they were to have (autism, asperger's syndrome, pervasive developmental disorder). In addition, indicate that they will be learning about something which could be called a *sixth sense,* and that they will be talking about ways to help someone who has difficulty with this sense.

Review of the senses: Ask the class to identify each of the following for each of the five senses:

1. Identify the sense/ is it learned or "automatic"?
2. Discuss how that sense helps us / how we use the sense/ what kind of information we receive through the sense
3. For sense of sight and hearing: Discuss what we know about people who have impairments in each of these area, and how to help them.

Write on the blackboard to record information as the discussion progresses, for example:

SIGHT: did anyone teach you to see?
- use sight to: know where we are going; learn; read, play, etc.
- to help people who are blind: use leader dogs, canes, other people to get around; braille; need things organized.

Demonstration of how "the sixth sense" works:
Tell the class you are going to show them how the sixth sense works. Ask for a volunteer, who remains seated. Select someone in the back half of the classroom. Ask that student to briefly describe things he/she sees, for example, the chalkboard, clock, etc.. Then, ask the student to identify things *you* see, for example, all the students and desks, the bulletin board display at the back of the room, etc.. Identify things you know are behind you (for example: chalkboard, clock), and ask the student if you can see them. Finally, ask the student how he/she did that - how was the student able to know what the room looks like from where you are standing? He/she will probably not know the answer, which is what you immediately provide. Explain that we all have this ability to imagine what things look, feel, and sound like to others - even if we are not right there with them. Ask the entire class: Did someone *TEACH* you to do that, or did you *"just know?"* Is *our ability to know what other people sense something we do automatically?* Record information on the chalkboard. For *younger* students, write:

We know what other people see, hear, taste, and touch.

For older students, explain we have the ability to take the *perceptual perspective* of others, we automatically know and keep track of what others are seeing, hearing, and sensing, and write:

> Perceptual perspective

Next, ask the students to watch as you hide a small object (stuffed animal). Ask a volunteer for his/her name (Adam) and ask Adam to leave the room. Establish everyone's attention as you *change the location of the stuffed animal* while Adam remains outside the room. Ask Adam to return to the classroom and to his/her seat.

Recruit a second volunteer (Jessica). Ask Jessica where *Adam thinks* the stuffed animal is located. Jessica should indicate the original, not the current, location. Explain that people keep track of what other people *know*. Did someone teach us to do that, or is it automatic, like our senses? For *younger students*, add to what is already on the chalkboard:

> *We know what other people see, hear, taste, and touch.*
>
> *We know what other people know.*

For older students, explain that we have the ability to keep track of what other people know, we can take what is called the *cognitive perspective* of others, and add to what is currently on the board:

> *Perceptual perspective*
>
> *Cognitive perspective*

Finally, explain that we also have the ability to know how people *feel*. Briefly discuss how we can tell how other people feel (facial expressions, how they move, what they say, how they say it, etc.). Add to the list (*for younger students*):

> *We know what other people see, hear, taste, and touch.*
>
> *We know what other people know.*
>
> *We know how other people feel.*

and review and title the list as *"The Sixth Sense: Our Social Sense":*

> *The Sixth Sense: Our Social Sense*
>
> *We know what other people see, hear, taste, and touch.*
>
> *We know what other people know.*
>
> *We know how other people feel.*

For older students, identify the ability to know what others feel as the ability to take the *affective perspective* of others. Explain that together the ability to take the perceptual, cognitive, and affective perspective make up what is called perspective taking ability. Title the completed list:

> *Perspective Taking Ability*
>
> *Perceptual perspective*
>
> *Cognitive perspective*
>
> *Affective perspective*

Discuss the social impairment: Quickly review what occurs when people are blind, or deaf. Explain that these people have impairments in their sense of sight and hearing, and need for others to understand. Ask students to imagine what it might be like to have an impaired social sense (or impairment in social cognition and perspective taking ability). If this is difficult for students to answer, guide their responses with questions like:

Would it be easy or difficult to take turns if you didn't know what others are thinking, or how they feel?

Would it be easy or difficult to talk to others about something they did?

Would it be easy or difficult to understand why we need rules for games?

Would it be easy or difficult to understand why people do things?

Would some things that people do take you by surprise? Might people frighten you sometimes?

Would it be easy or difficult to make friends?

Explain that the included classmate may have difficulty with these things.

Conclusion: ***Identify student solutions:*** Ask the students to identify how they might assist their classmate. Write their ideas on the board. Students may need help with this, incorporate your understanding of the individual included student to guide the students in identifying ways they can assist their classmate.

Socially Simplifying a Playground
with a Piece of Chalk
- Carol Gray
Consultant to Students with Autism

Helping students with autism to interact effectively with others is an ongoing priority. On a playground during recess, the challenge to students with autism can be overwhelming. The ideas on this sheet require blacktop and a piece of chalk, and are meant to be used along with other materials and supports to help students with autism be more successful at recess.

Help with Standing in Line

Using chalk, draw a rectangle for the student to go to when the bell rings - other children can line up at random on either side. Variations: 1) Write the student's name in the rectangle; 2) Write a cue for a desired behavior, for example: FACE THIS WAY or WAIT FOR DIRECTIONS FROM THE TEACHER, etc; or 3) use a broken line to identify the rectangle to make it easier to fade if possible.

Help with Taking Turns

These ideas require the cooperation of a group of children - general education students often find these modifications very helpful to them, as well. Any number of possibilities exist, here are a few:

1. For a game played in a given area, or for several children waiting to play with a given piece of equipment which requires turn taking: Children "sign in", writing their names in a list with a piece of chalk. Children follow the list to take turns. A child may serve as "director" - moving from one name to another to announce whose turn is next.

2. For shooting baskets: Draw spaces in an arc, like pictured below. Students each stand in a space, taking turns in a row at shooting the basket. When the ball reaches the last child, the ball is passed back to the child in the starting space, and the children rotate one space to the right to take turns shooting from a new position. One school had the idea to make these lines permanent, with white paint.

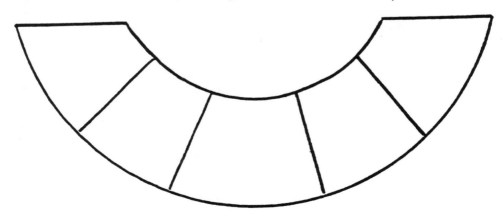

<u>Help with Communication</u> "I want to be alone for awhile."

Identify a space on the playground with chalk, and teach the student and other children that it is the student's "space".

<u>Other Ideas</u>

Ask the student or other children for ideas of "what to write" - or other ideas to structure games so they run more smoothly. The possibilities are literally endless, the goal is to provide a visual sense of structure to a situation which can be otherwise overwhelming. Have fun!

Sample Recess Social Story

The following story "It's Time for Recess", by Carol Gray, is a sample of a social story written for a first grade boy with autism who was fearful of going out to recess. The story was successful in assisting him in understanding the variety of activities at recess, and he was going out to recess a few days after the story was first introduced.

This story is intended to be used as a sample for other possible recess social stories. The stories you write will reflect the factors influencing your individual student and situation. For example, photographs are not necessary for a social story to be effective. Sometimes, stories are written without the use of pictures or illustrations, or with stick figures which accompany the story.

Additional materials describing how to write and implement social stories are available at cost from: **FUTURE HORIZONS** ɪɴᴄ. **424 Lamar Blvd. East, Arlington, TX 76011. (817) 277-0727. FAX: (817) 277-2270.**

I go to Lincoln School. I am in Mrs. Johnson's kindergarten class.

Almost every day we go outside for recess. Sometimes when it is cold, I put on my jacket and hat.   This is a picture I drew of me in my coat and hat. I'm ready for recess!

There are many children at recess. There are many things to play with, too! Some children run to the slide. Some children like the cross bars. Some children like to climb the monkey bars. Each child tries to find something fun to do.

The slide is very tall. Some children climb the stairs to the very top. But the best part is S
                              L
                                 I
                                  D
                                     I
                                        N
                                          G

down! Wow, that is pretty fast!

Sometimes there is a line of children waiting for a turn on the slide. If I get in the line, soon I will be FIRST. We all have to wait to be FIRST so we can take our turn. Then we slide down!

Some boys are great climbers. They start at the very bottom and crawl to the top. They hold on tight and move very slowly. Children move slowly when they climb to be sure their feet and hands are in the right place. Many children think it's fun to climb, and to look at everyone from the top.

Many children think the bars are fun. When children have fun, sometimes they smile.

Some children take a ball out to recess. I can roll it, toss it, catch it, throw it,

           e
or b   c   it. If I find a friend who also wants to play, they can
    o n
      u

         e
b   c   it back to them. I can roll the ball. Balls may be fun at recess
  o n
    u

There are also friends to play with at recess. It might be fun to be with a friend on the playground.

If I want, I can talk to the teacher on the playground. Usually, teachers are very nice. A teacher can help me if I have a problem. I can go up and talk with a teacher at recess.

The bell rings to tell us when recess is over. We get into line to go back to class. Once we are in class, the playground is very quiet. All the children are inside.